WEIGHT LOSS DIET COOKBOOK FOR WOMEN

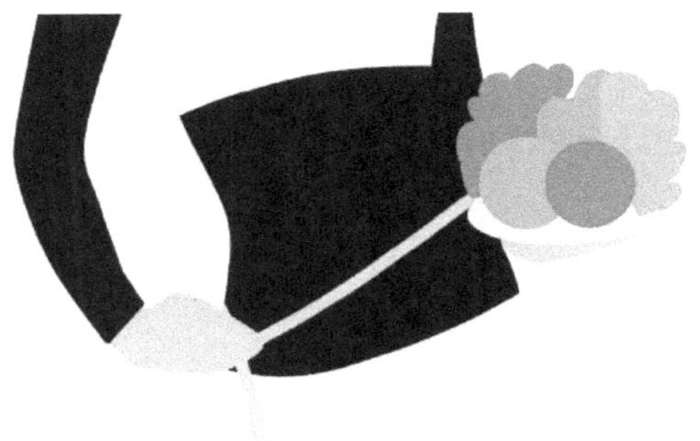

Delicious, Nutrient-rich Diet Recipes and Expert Advice for Women Seeking Quick, Healthy Weight Loss

Scott C. Horvath

Copyright © 2024 by Scott C. Horvath

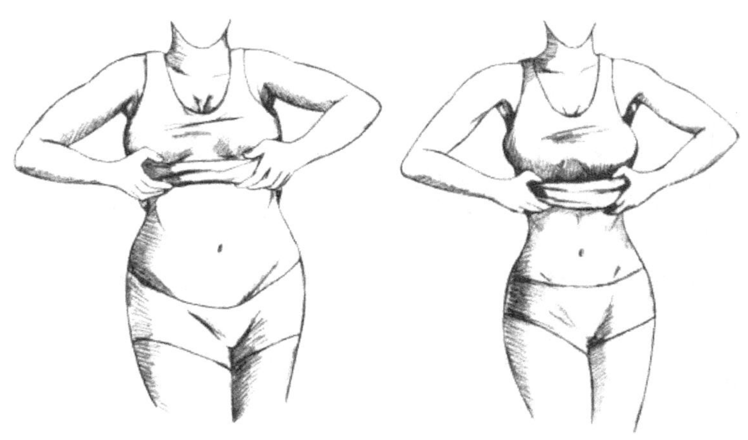

INTRODUCTION

Olivia had always struggled with her weight. No matter how hard she tried, the pounds just wouldn't budge. She had tried every diet out there, from low-carb to high-protein, but nothing seemed to work. Frustrated and disheartened, she was about to give up when she stumbled upon a link to **Weight Loss Diet Cookbook for Women** on social media promising a solution.

Intrigued, Olivia clicked on the link and found herself on a website promoting the cookbook. As she scrolled through the page, she was impressed by the testimonials of women who had successfully lost weight using the recipes. With a glimmer of hope, Olivia decided to give it a try and purchased the cookbook.

As soon as the cookbook arrived, Olivia eagerly flipped through the pages, marveling at the mouthwatering recipes. She couldn't believe that she could eat such delicious food and still lose weight. Excited, she headed to the grocery store to stock up on ingredients.

For the next few weeks, Olivia threw herself into her new diet, preparing meals from the cookbook every day. She couldn't believe how easy it was to stick to the plan. Not only were the recipes delicious, but they were also quick and easy to make, perfect for her busy lifestyle.

Before long, Olivia started to notice a difference. The pounds were melting away, and she had more energy than ever before. For the first time in years, she felt happy and healthier.

When she stepped on the scale and saw that she had lost ten pounds, Olivia couldn't contain her excitement. She knew that she had finally found the solution she had been searching for.

Thanks to the **Weight Loss Diet Cookbook for Women** she found through that social media link, Olivia was able to achieve her weight loss goals and transform her life. She couldn't wait to see what other delicious recipes awaited her in its pages.

In a world where fitness and health are becoming increasingly important, weight loss has become a common goal for many individuals.

Whether it's for health reasons, to boost confidence, or simply to feel better, shedding excess weight is a journey that requires dedication, patience, and the right approach.

Understanding Weight Loss

Weight loss is more than just about shedding a few pounds; it's about adopting a healthier lifestyle. While crash diets and intense workout regimens might promise quick results, sustainable weight loss is a gradual process that involves making long-term changes to your eating habits, physical activity levels, and overall mindset.

Importance of Healthy Weight Loss

Maintaining a healthy weight is crucial for overall well-being. Excess weight can increase the risk of various health problems, including heart disease, diabetes, and joint pain. By losing weight in a healthy and sustainable manner, you not only improve your physical health but also boost your mental and emotional well-being.

Key Principles of Weight Loss

Balanced Diet: A healthy, balanced diet is the foundation of any successful weight loss journey. Focus on incorporating plenty of fruits, vegetables, lean proteins, and whole grains into your meals while limiting processed foods, sugary snacks, and high-calorie beverages.

Regular Exercise: Physical activity is essential for burning calories, building muscle, and boosting metabolism. Aim for at least 150 minutes of moderate-intensity exercise or 75 minutes of vigorous-intensity exercise each week, along with strength training exercises at least two days a week.

Lifestyle Changes: Sustainable weight loss requires long-term lifestyle changes. This includes getting enough sleep, managing stress, staying hydrated, and practicing mindful eating.

Setting Realistic Goals: Set achievable, realistic goals for yourself. Aim for gradual weight loss of 1-2 pounds per week, as this is more likely to lead to long-term success.

Embarking on a weight loss journey can be challenging, but it's also incredibly rewarding. By making healthier choices, staying committed, and seeking support when needed, you can achieve your weight loss goals and improve your overall quality of life. Remember, it's not just about losing weight; it's about becoming the healthiest and happiest version of yourself.

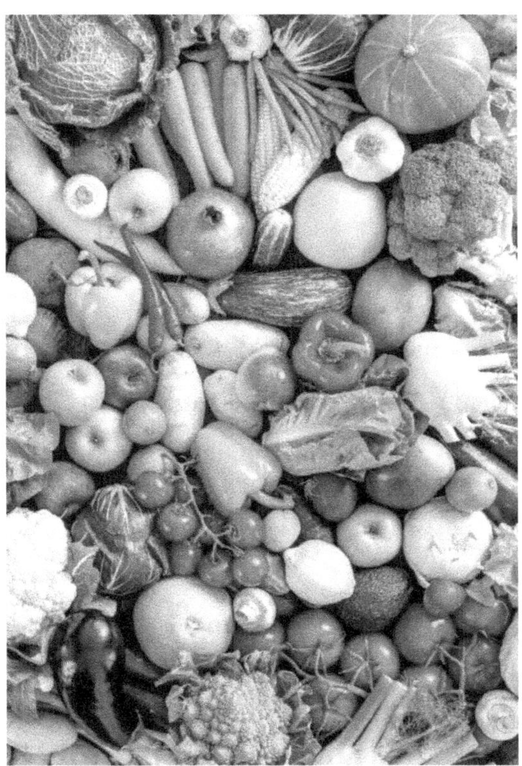

CHAPTER 1

Understanding Weight Loss

In a world where fitness and health are becoming increasingly important, weight loss has become a common goal for many individuals. Whether it's for health reasons, to boost confidence, or simply to feel better, shedding excess weight is a journey that requires dedication, patience, and the right approach.

The Science behind Weight Loss

Weight loss is more than just about shedding a few pounds; it's about adopting a healthier lifestyle. At its core, weight loss is a result of burning more calories than you consume. This is achieved through a combination of diet, exercise, and lifestyle changes.

Caloric Deficit: To lose weight, you need to create a caloric deficit, which means burning more calories than you consume. You can accomplish this by cutting calories, upping your physical activity, or doing both at once.

Metabolism: Your metabolism plays a crucial role in weight loss. Your body uses this process to turn food into energy. Factors such as age, gender, body composition, and activity level all influence your metabolism.

Nutrition: A balanced diet is essential for weight loss. Make a point of eating full, nutrient-dense foods like whole grains, fruits, and vegetables as well as lean proteins. These foods give you vital nutrients and make you feel content and full.

Physical Activity: Regular exercise is key to weight loss. It not only burns calories but also helps build muscle, boost metabolism, and improve overall health. Try to incorporate cardiovascular, strength, and flexibility training into your routine.

Setting Realistic Goals

For a weight loss journey to be successful, setting reasonable goals is crucial. How to position yourself for success is as follows:

Be Specific: Set clear, specific goals for yourself. Instead of saying, "I want to lose weight," try setting a specific target, such as "I want to lose 10 pounds in the next two months."

Be Realistic: Set achievable goals that you can realistically reach. Aim for a gradual weight loss of 1-2 pounds per week, as this is more sustainable in the long run.

Focus on Health: Instead of focusing solely on the number on the scale, focus on improving your overall health and well-being. Appreciate non-scale accomplishments like more energy, a happier attitude, and better sleep.

Track Your Progress: Keep track of your progress by recording your food intake, exercise routine, and measurements. This will enable you to maintain accountability and make changes as necessary.

While starting a weight loss journey can be difficult, it can also be quite rewarding. By understanding the science behind weight loss, setting realistic goals, and making healthy lifestyle changes, you can achieve your weight loss goals and improve your overall quality of life. Remember, it's not just about losing weight; it's about becoming the healthiest and happiest version of yourself.

CHAPTER 2

Understanding the Cause of Weight Gain

Weight gain is a complex process influenced by various factors, including genetics, metabolism, environment, and lifestyle. By understanding the underlying causes of weight gain, you can take proactive steps to manage your weight effectively.

Calorie Imbalance: Weight gain often occurs when there is an imbalance between the number of calories consumed and the number of calories burned. Consuming more calories than your body needs for energy leads to excess weight storage in the form of fat.

Unhealthy Eating Habits: Poor dietary choices, such as consuming high-calorie, low-nutrient foods, can contribute to weight gain. Processed foods, sugary snacks, and high-fat meals are often calorie-dense and lacking in essential nutrients, leading to overeating and weight gain.

Sedentary Lifestyle: Lack of physical activity is a significant contributor to weight gain. Inactivity not only burns fewer calories but also leads to loss of muscle mass and a slower metabolism, making it easier to gain weight and harder to lose it.

Genetics: Genetic factors can play a role in determining a person's susceptibility to weight gain. While genetics may predispose some individuals to gain weight more easily than others, lifestyle factors such as diet and exercise still play a significant role in managing weight.

Hormonal Imbalance: Hormonal changes can affect metabolism, appetite, and fat storage, leading to weight gain. Conditions such as hypothyroidism, insulin resistance, and polycystic ovary syndrome (PCOS) can disrupt hormonal balance and contribute to weight gain.

Stress and Emotional Eating: Stress, anxiety, and other emotional factors can lead to overeating and weight gain. Many people turn to food for comfort during times of stress, which can lead to a pattern of emotional eating and unhealthy weight gain.

Lack of Sleep: Sleep plays a crucial role in regulating appetite hormones and metabolism. Chronic sleep deprivation can disrupt these hormones, leading to increased appetite, cravings for high-calorie foods, and weight gain.

Understanding the causes of weight gain is the first step towards effectively managing and maintaining a healthy weight.

By addressing unhealthy eating habits, increasing physical activity, managing stress, and prioritizing adequate sleep, you can take control of your weight and improve your overall health and well-being. Remember, small changes add up over time, and adopting a healthy lifestyle is the key to long-term weight management.

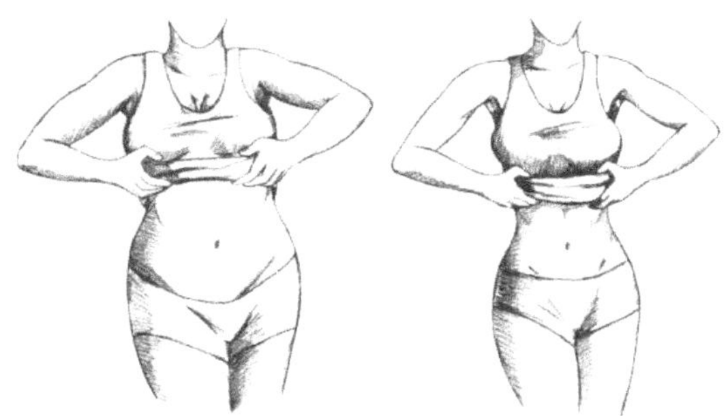

CHAPTER 3

Building Healthy Eating Habits

When it comes to losing weight and improving your overall health, building healthy eating habits is essential. Rather than focusing on short-term diets, adopting a sustainable approach to eating can lead to long-lasting results. Here are two key components to building healthy eating habits:

Balancing Macronutrients

Macronutrients are the fundamental components of a balanced diet, and they include lipids, proteins, and carbs. Balancing these nutrients is crucial for providing your body with the energy and nutrients it needs to function optimally. Carbohydrates: Choose complex carbohydrates such as whole grains, fruits, and vegetables over simple carbohydrates like sugary snacks and refined grains. Complex carbohydrates provide sustained energy and are rich in essential nutrients and fiber.

Proteins: Incorporate lean sources of protein into your meals, such as chicken, turkey, fish, tofu, beans, and legumes. Protein helps to keep you feeling full and satisfied, supports muscle growth and repair, and helps to stabilize blood sugar levels.

Fats: Choose the healthy fats that are present in foods like olive oil, avocados, almonds, and seeds. These fats are essential for brain function, hormone production, and the absorption of fat-soluble vitamins.

Smart Snacking

Smart snacking can help you stay satisfied between meals and prevent overeating. Choose nutrient-dense snacks that provide a combination of protein, healthy fats, and fiber to keep you feeling full and energized.

Fruit and Nut Butter: Pairing a piece of fruit with a tablespoon of nut butter provides a satisfying combination of carbohydrates, protein, and healthy fats.

Berries with Greek Yogurt: Berries offer natural sweetness and fiber, while Greek yogurt is high in calcium and protein.

Vegetable Sticks with Hummus: Crunchy vegetables like carrots, cucumber, and bell peppers paired with hummus make for a satisfying and nutritious snack.

Whole Grain Crackers with Cheese: The cheese contributes calcium and protein, while the whole grain crackers offer fiber and complex carbs.

By focusing on balanced meals and smart snacking, you can build healthy eating habits that support your weight loss and overall health goals. Remember to listen to your body, eat mindfully, and make choices that nourish and energize you.

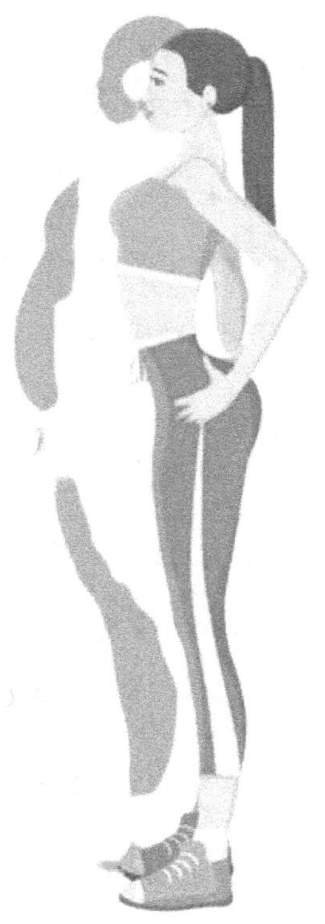

CHAPTER 4

Weight loss meal plan for women

Day 1

Breakfast: Greek yogurt topped with chia seeds and a mixture of berries.

Dessert: Carrot sticks with hummus.

Lunch: mixed greens, cucumber, cherry tomatoes, and balsamic vinaigrette topped with grilled chicken salad.

Dessert: Apple slices with almond butter.

Dinner: baked salmon served over quinoa and steaming broccoli.

Day 2

- **Breakfast**: Banana slices and honey drizzled over oatmeal.

- **Dessert**: Handful of almonds.

- **Lunch**: Wrap with avocado and turkey on a whole grain tortilla.

- **Snack**: Greek yogurt with sliced strawberries.

- **Dinner**: Brown rice is served with stir-fried tofu and a mixture of veggies.

Day 3

- **Breakfast**: Poached egg, smashed avocado, and whole grain bread.

- **Dessert**: Celery sticks with peanut butter.

- **Lunch**: Quinoa salad with black beans, corn, bell peppers, and a squeeze of lime juice.

- **Dessert**: Cottage cheese with pineapple chunks.

- **Dinner**: grilled shrimp served with sweet potato and roasted asparagus.

Day 4:

- **Breakfast**: Omelet of spinach and feta served with whole grain bread on the side.

- **Dessert**: Mixed berries.

- **Lunch**: Curry made with beans and vegetables and served over brown rice.

- **Dessert**: Cherry tomatoes with mozzarella cheese.

- **Dinner**: roasted Brussels sprouts, baked chicken breast, and a side salad.

Day 5:

- **Breakfast**: Smoothie made with spinach, banana, frozen berries, and almond milk.

- **Dessert**: Edamame beans.

- **Lunch**: Tuna salad made with Greek yogurt, celery, and onions, served on whole grain crackers.

- **Dessert**: Orange slices.

- **Dinner**: Marinara sauce and zucchini noodles paired with turkey meatballs.

Day 6

Breakfast: Peach slices and a dash of cinnamon over cottage cheese.
- **Dessert**: Avocado slices on top of rice cakes.
- **Lunch**: Lentil soup and mixed green salad.
- **Dessert**: A few walnuts mixed with slices of pears.
- **Dinner**: Baked cod over quinoa and steamed green beans.

Day 7

- **Breakfast**: Whole grain waffle with mixed berries and Greek yogurt.
- **Dessert**: Hummus-topped baby carrots.
- **Lunch**: Salad of grilled vegetables and feta cheese drizzled with balsamic glaze.

- **Dessert**: A handful of grapes as a snack.
- **Dessert**: Brown rice with a stir-fried beef dish that includes broccoli, bell peppers, and snap peas.
Always remember to stay hydrated throughout the day and modify portion sizes based on your caloric needs.

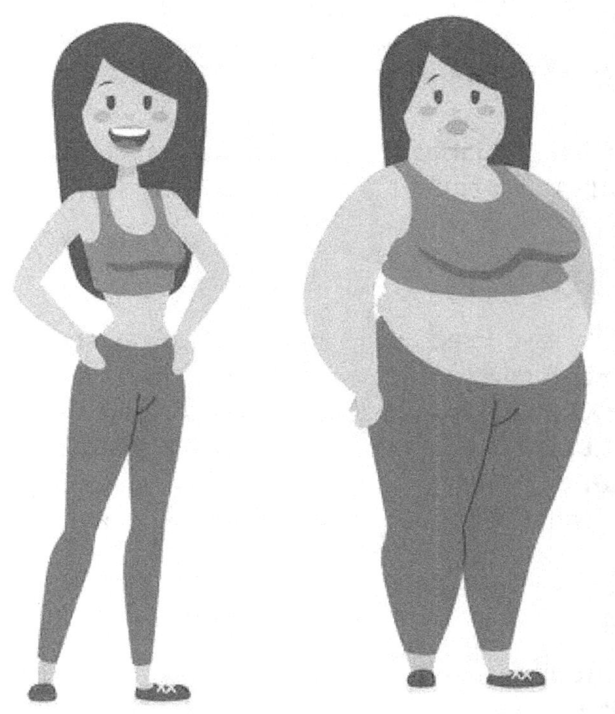

CHAPTER 5

10-day weight loss meal plan for women

Day 1

Breakfast: Avocado and Egg Toast

Ingredients:

- 1 slice whole grain bread

- 1/2 avocado, mashed

- 1 egg, poached or fried

- Salt and pepper to taste

Instructions:

1. Toast the whole grain bread until golden brown.

2. Spread the mashed avocado over the toast.

3. Top with a poached or fried egg.

4. Season with salt and pepper to taste.

Lunch: Grilled Chicken Salad

Ingredients:

- 100g grilled chicken breast, sliced

- Mixed salad greens

- Cherry tomatoes, halved

- Cucumber, sliced

- Balsamic vinaigrette

Instructions:

1. Arrange the mixed salad greens, cherry tomatoes, and cucumber on a plate.

2. Top with sliced grilled chicken breast.

3. Drizzle with balsamic vinaigrette.

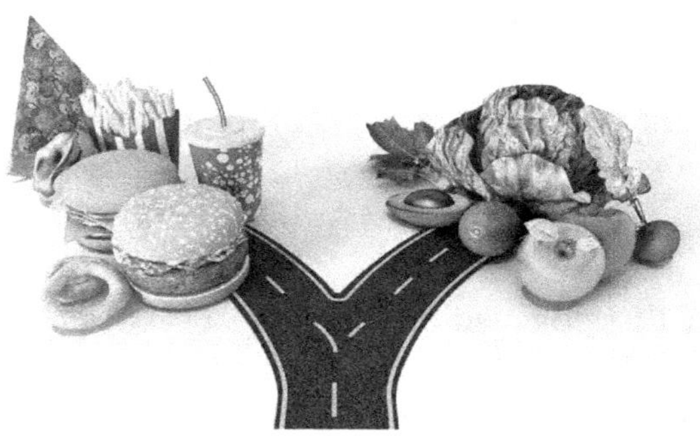

Dinner: Baked Salmon with Steamed Broccoli and Quinoa

Ingredients:

- 1 salmon fillet

- 1/2 cup quinoa

- 1 cup broccoli florets

- Lemon slices

- Olive oil

- Salt and pepper to taste

Instructions:

1. Preheat the oven to 375°F (190°C).

2. Season the salmon fillet with salt, pepper, and a drizzle of olive oil. Place lemon slices on top.

3. Bake the salmon for 15-20 minutes until cooked through.

4. Meanwhile, cook the quinoa according to package instructions.

5. Steam the broccoli until tender.

6. Serve the baked salmon with steamed broccoli and quinoa.

Day 2

Breakfast:

Greek Yogurt with Mixed Berries and Chia Seeds

Ingredients:

- 1/2 cup Greek yogurt

- Mixed berries (strawberries, blueberries, raspberries)

- 1 tablespoon chia seeds

Instructions:

1. In a bowl, add Greek yogurt.

2. Top with mixed berries and sprinkle chia seeds over the top.

Lunch:
Turkey and Avocado Wrap
- Ingredients:

- 100g sliced turkey breast

- 1 whole grain tortilla

- 1/4 avocado, sliced

- Lettuce leaves

- Tomato slices

- Instructions:

1. Lay the whole-grain tortilla flat.

2. Layer sliced turkey breast, avocado, lettuce, and tomato on the tortilla.

3. Roll up the tortilla and cut in half.

Dinner: Stir-fried tofu with Mixed Vegetables over Brown Rice

- Ingredients:

- 150g firm tofu, cubed

- Assorted mixed vegetables (bell peppers, broccoli, carrots, snap peas)

- 1 cup cooked brown rice

- Soy sauce

- Garlic powder

- Sesame oil

Instructions:

1. Heat sesame oil in a pan over medium heat.

2. Add cubed tofu and stir-fry until golden brown.

3. Add mixed vegetables and continue to stir-fry until vegetables are tender.

4. Season with garlic powder and soy sauce.

5. Serve over cooked brown rice.

Day 3

Breakfast: Spinach and Feta Omelet

Ingredients:

- 2 eggs

- Handful of spinach leaves

- 2 tablespoons crumbled feta cheese

- Salt and pepper to taste

Instructions:

1. In a bowl, beat the eggs and season with salt and pepper.

2. Heat a non-stick skillet over medium heat and add the beaten eggs.

3. Once the eggs start to set, add spinach leaves and feta cheese to one side of the omelet.

4. Fold the omelet in half and cook until the cheese is melted and the eggs are cooked through.

Lunch: Quinoa Salad with Black Beans, Corn, and Bell Peppers

- Ingredients:

- 1/2 cup cooked quinoa

- 1/4 cup black beans, drained and rinsed

- 1/4 cup corn kernels

- 1/4 cup diced bell peppers

- Fresh cilantro, chopped

- Lime juice

- Salt and pepper to taste

- Instructions:

1. In a bowl, combine cooked quinoa, black beans, corn, bell peppers, and cilantro.

2. Squeeze fresh lime juice over the salad and season with salt and pepper.

Dinner: Grilled Shrimp with Roasted Asparagus and Sweet Potato

Ingredients:

- 100g shrimp, peeled and deveined

- 1 sweet potato, sliced

- 1 bunch asparagus, trimmed

- Olive oil

- Garlic powder

- Paprika

- Salt and pepper to taste

Instructions:

1. Preheat the oven to 400°F (200°C).

2. Place sweet potato slices and asparagus on a baking sheet.

3. Drizzle with olive oil and season with garlic powder, paprika, salt, and pepper.

4. Roast in the oven for 20-25 minutes until tender.

5. Meanwhile, grill the shrimp until cooked through.

6. Serve grilled shrimp with roasted asparagus and sweet potato slices.

Day 4:

Breakfast: Overnight Oats with Mixed Berries

Ingredients:

- 1/2 cup rolled oats

- 1/2 cup unsweetened almond milk

- 1/4 cup Greek yogurt

- Mixed berries (strawberries, blueberries, raspberries)

- 1 tablespoon honey or maple syrup (optional)

Instructions:

1. In a jar or bowl, combine rolled oats, almond milk, Greek yogurt, and honey or maple syrup (if using).

2. Stir well, then cover and refrigerate overnight.

3. In the morning, top with mixed berries before serving.

Lunch: Tuna Salad on Whole Grain Crackers

Ingredients:

- 1 can tuna, drained

- 2 tablespoons Greek yogurt

- 1 tablespoon chopped celery

- 1 tablespoon chopped red onion

- Salt and pepper to taste

- Whole grain crackers

Instructions:

1. In a bowl, combine tuna, Greek yogurt, celery, red onion, salt, and pepper.

2. Mix until well combined.

3. Serve tuna salad on top of whole grain crackers.

Dinner:

Beef Stir-Fry with Broccoli and Bell Peppers served over Brown Rice

- Ingredients:

- 100g beef strips

- Assorted mixed vegetables (broccoli, bell peppers, carrots)

- 1 cup cooked brown rice

- Soy sauce

- Garlic powder

- Sesame oil

Instructions:

1. Heat sesame oil in a pan over medium heat.

2. Add beef strips and stir-fry until browned.

3. Add mixed vegetables and continue to stir-fry until vegetables are tender.

4. Season with garlic powder and soy sauce.

5. Serve over cooked brown rice.

Day 5

Breakfast: Mixed Berry Smoothie

Ingredients:

- 1/2 cup mixed berries (strawberries, blueberries, raspberries)

- 1/2 banana

- 1/2 cup spinach leaves

- 1/2 cup unsweetened almond milk

- 1 tablespoon chia seeds

Instructions:

1. Place all ingredients in a blender.

2. Blend until smooth and creamy.

3. Pour into a glass and serve immediately.

Lunch: Lentil Soup

- Ingredients:

- 1/2 cup lentils, rinsed and drained

- 1 carrot, diced

- 1 celery stalk, diced

- 1/2 onion, diced

- 2 cups vegetable broth

- Salt and pepper to taste

Instructions:

1. In a pot, combine lentils, carrot, celery, onion, and vegetable broth.

2. Bring to a boil, then reduce heat and simmer for 20-25 minutes until lentils are tender.

3. Season with salt and pepper to taste.

Dinner: Turkey Meatballs with Zucchini Noodles and Marinara Sauce

- Ingredients:

- 100g ground turkey

- 1/4 cup breadcrumbs

- 1 egg

- 1/2 teaspoon garlic powder

- 1/2 teaspoon dried oregano

- Salt and pepper to taste

- 1 zucchini, paralyzed into noodles

- Marinara sauce

Instructions:

1. Preheat the oven to 375°F (190°C).

2. In a bowl, combine ground turkey, breadcrumbs, egg, garlic powder, oregano, salt, and pepper. Mix until well combined.

3. Roll the mixture into meatballs and place on a baking sheet.

4. Bake for 20-25 minutes until cooked through.

5. Meanwhile, sauté zucchini noodles in a pan until tender.

6. Serve turkey meatballs with zucchini noodles and marinara sauce.

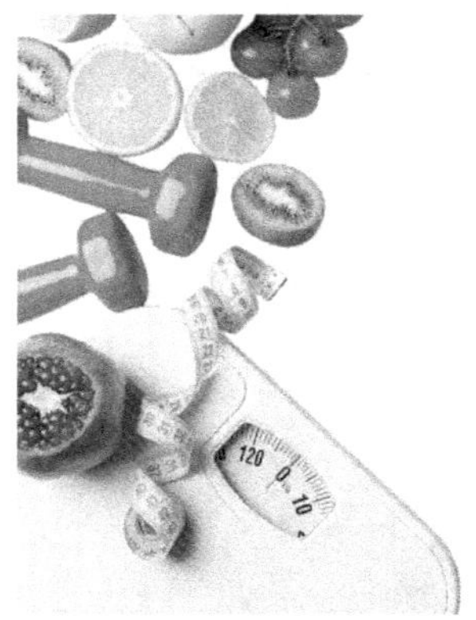

Day 6

Breakfast: Cottage Cheese with Peaches and Cinnamon

Ingredients:

- 1/2 cup cottage cheese

- 1 peach, sliced

- Pinch of cinnamon

- Instructions:

1. In a bowl, add cottage cheese.

2. Top with sliced peaches.

3. Sprinkle with cinnamon.

Lunch: Turkey and Hummus Wrap

- Ingredients:

- 100g sliced turkey breast

- 1 whole grain tortilla

- 2 tablespoons hummus

- Mixed salad greens

- Tomato slices

Instructions:

1. Lay the whole grain tortilla flat.

2. Spread hummus over the tortilla.

3. Layer sliced turkey breast, mixed salad greens, and tomato slices on top.

4. Roll up the tortilla and cut in half.

Dinner: Baked Cod with Steamed Green Beans and Quinoa

Ingredients:

- 1 cod fillet

- 1/2 cup quinoa

- 1 cup green beans, trimmed

- Lemon slices

- Olive oil

- Salt and pepper to taste

Instructions:

1. Preheat the oven to 375°F (190°C).

2. Season the cod fillet with salt, pepper, and a drizzle of olive oil. Place lemon slices on top.

3. Bake the cod for 15-20 minutes until cooked through.

4. Meanwhile, cook the quinoa according to package instructions.

5. Steam the green beans until tender.

6. Serve the baked cod with steamed green beans and quinoa.

Day 7

Breakfast: Whole Grain Waffle with Greek Yogurt and Mixed Berries

Ingredients:

- 1 whole grain waffle

- 1/4 cup Greek yogurt

- Mixed berries (strawberries, blueberries, raspberries)

Instructions:

1. Toast the whole grain waffle until golden brown.

2. Top with Greek yogurt and mixed berries.

Lunch: Grilled Vegetable and Feta Cheese Salad

- Ingredients:

- Assorted mixed greens

- Grilled vegetables (bell peppers, zucchini, eggplant)

- 2 tablespoons crumbled feta cheese

- Balsamic glaze

Instructions:

1. Arrange mixed greens on a plate.

2. Top with grilled vegetables and crumbled feta cheese.

3. Drizzle with balsamic glaze.

Dinner: Beef Stir-Fry with Snow Peas and Brown Rice

- Ingredients:

- 100g beef strips

- 1 cup snow peas

- 1/2 cup sliced carrots

- 1/2 cup sliced bell peppers

- 1 cup cooked brown rice

- Soy sauce

- Garlic powder

- Sesame oil

Instructions:

1. Heat sesame oil in a pan over medium heat.

2. Add beef strips and stir-fry until browned.

3. Add snow peas, carrots, and bell peppers and continue to stir-fry until vegetables are tender.

4. Season with garlic powder and soy sauce.

5. Serve over cooked brown rice.

Day 8:

Breakfast: Banana and Peanut Butter Smoothie

Ingredients:

- 1 banana

- 1 tablespoon peanut butter

- 1/2 cup unsweetened almond milk

- 1/2 cup Greek yogurt

- Handful of spinach (optional)

Instructions:

1. Combine all ingredients in a blender.

2. Blend until smooth.

3. Pour into a glass and serve immediately.

Lunch: Chickpea and Avocado Salad

Ingredients:

- 1/2 cup chickpeas, drained and rinsed

- 1/4 avocado, diced

- Mixed salad greens

- Cherry tomatoes, halved

- Cucumber slices

- Lemon vinaigrette

Instructions:

1. In a bowl, combine chickpeas, avocado, mixed salad greens, cherry tomatoes, and cucumber.

2. Drizzle with lemon vinaigrette.

Dinner: Grilled Chicken with Roasted Brussels Sprouts and Sweet Potato

Ingredients:

- 1 chicken breast

- 1 cup Brussels sprouts, halved

- 1 sweet potato, diced

- Olive oil

- Garlic powder

- Paprika

- Salt and pepper to taste

Instructions:

1. Preheat the oven to 400°F (200°C).

2. Season the chicken breast with garlic powder, paprika, salt, and pepper.

3. Place the chicken breast on a baking sheet.

4. Toss Brussels sprouts and sweet potato with olive oil, garlic powder, salt, and pepper.

5. Arrange Brussels sprouts and sweet potato on the baking sheet around the chicken breast.

6. Bake for 20-25 minutes until the chicken is cooked through and the vegetables are tender.

Day 9:

Breakfast: Quinoa Breakfast Bowl

Ingredients:

- 1/2 cup cooked quinoa

- 1/4 cup Greek yogurt

- Mixed berries (strawberries, blueberries, raspberries)

- 1 tablespoon honey or maple syrup (optional)

Instructions:

1. In a bowl, layer cooked quinoa, Greek yogurt, and mixed berries.

2. Drizzle with honey or maple syrup if desired.

Lunch: Caprese Salad

Ingredients:

- Fresh mozzarella cheese, sliced

- Tomato, sliced

- Fresh basil leaves

- Balsamic glaze

Instructions:

1. Arrange sliced mozzarella cheese, tomato, and basil leaves on a plate.

2. Drizzle with balsamic glaze.

Dinner: Baked Tilapia with Sautéed Spinach and Brown Rice

Ingredients:

- 1 tilapia fillet

- 2 cups fresh spinach

- 1 garlic clove, minced

- Olive oil

- Lemon juice

- Salt and pepper to taste

- 1 cup cooked brown rice

Instructions:

1. Preheat the oven to 375°F (190°C).

2. Place the tilapia fillet on a baking sheet.

3. Drizzle with olive oil and lemon juice. Season with salt and pepper.

4. Bake for 15-20 minutes until the fish is cooked through.

5. Meanwhile, heat olive oil in a pan over medium heat.

6. Add minced garlic and sauté until fragrant.

7. Add fresh spinach and sauté until wilted.

8. Serve baked tilapia with sautéed spinach and brown rice.

Day 10:

Breakfast: Veggie Omelet

Ingredients:

- 2 eggs

- Assorted mixed vegetables (bell peppers, onions, spinach, mushrooms)

- Olive oil

- Salt and pepper to taste

Instructions:

1. In a bowl, beat the eggs and season with salt and pepper.

2. Heat olive oil in a non-stick skillet over medium heat.

3. Add mixed vegetables and sauté until tender.

4. Pour beaten eggs over the vegetables and cook until set.

5. Fold the omelet in half and serve.

Lunch: Turkey and Quinoa Stuffed Bell Peppers

Ingredients:

- 2 bell peppers, halved and seeds removed

- 100g ground turkey

- 1/2 cup cooked quinoa

- 1/4 cup diced tomatoes

- 1/4 cup black beans, drained and rinsed

- 1/4 teaspoon chili powder

- 1/4 teaspoon cumin

- Salt and pepper to taste

Instructions:

1. Preheat the oven to 375°F (190°C).

2. In a skillet, cook ground turkey until browned.

3. Add diced tomatoes, cooked quinoa, black beans, chili powder, cumin, salt, and pepper. Cook for 5 minutes.

4. Stuff bell pepper halves with the turkey and quinoa mixture.

5. Place stuffed bell peppers on a baking sheet and bake for 20-25 minutes until peppers are tender.

Dinner: Grilled Salmon with Steamed Asparagus and Quinoa

Ingredients:

- 1 salmon fillet

- 1 cup asparagus spears, trimmed

- 1/2 cup cooked quinoa

- Lemon slices

- Olive oil

- Salt and pepper to taste

Instructions:

1. Preheat the grill to medium-high heat.

2. Season the salmon fillet with salt, pepper, and a drizzle of olive oil. Place lemon slices on top.

3. Grill the salmon for 4-5 minutes per side until cooked through.

4. Meanwhile, steam the asparagus until tender.

5. Serve grilled salmon with steamed asparagus and quinoa.

This 10-day meal plan provides a variety of delicious and nutritious recipes to help support your weight loss goals. Enjoy!

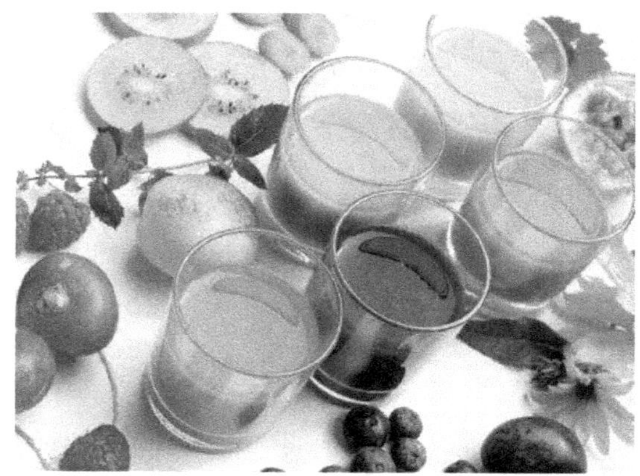

CHAPTER 6

Exercise and Movement Suitable for Women

Warm-up (5-10 minutes)

Jumping Jacks: 1 minute

Arm Circles: 30 seconds forward, 30 seconds backward

Bodyweight Squats: 1 minute

Hip Circles: 30 seconds in each direction

Torso Twists: 1 minute

Cardiovascular Exercise (20-30 minutes)

Choose one or a combination of the following:

Brisk Walking or Jogging: 20-30 minutes

Cycling: 20-30 minutes

Swimming: 20-30 minutes

Jump Rope: 10-15 minutes

Dancing: 20-30 minutes

Strength Training (20-30 minutes)

Perform each exercise for 2-3 sets of 10-12 repetitions:

Bodyweight Squats

Lunges (alternating legs)

Push-ups (can be done on knees if needed)

Dumbbell Rows (use water bottles or light dumbbells)

Dumbbell Shoulder Press (use water bottles or light dumbbells)

Bicep Curls (use water bottles or light dumbbells)

Triceps Dips (use a sturdy chair)

Plank (hold for 30-60 seconds)

Russian Twists (with or without weight)

Flexibility and Cool Down (5-10 minutes)

Hamstring Stretch: Hold for 30 seconds on each leg

Quad Stretch: Hold for 30 seconds on each leg

Calf Stretch: Hold for 30 seconds on each leg

Triceps Stretch: Hold for 30 seconds on each arm

Chest Stretch: Hold for 30 seconds

Shoulder Stretch: Hold for 30 seconds on each arm

Child's Pose: Hold for 1 minute

Seated Forward Bend: Hold for 1 minute

Cat-Cow Stretch: 1 minute

Additional Tips:

Hydration: Drink plenty of water before, during, and after exercise.

Nutrition: Maintain a balanced diet with a focus on lean proteins, vegetables, fruits, and whole grains.

Rest: Ensure you get enough rest and sleep for muscle recovery.

Consistency: Aim for at least 3-5 days of exercise per week.

Progression: Gradually increase the intensity or duration of your workouts as your fitness improves.

Incorporate HIIT (High-Intensity Interval Training: Integrate short bursts of intense exercise with periods of rest to maximize calorie burn in less time.

Include Core Work: Add exercises that target the core such as crunches, bicycle crunches, and leg raises to strengthen the abdominal muscles.

Mind-Body Exercises: Consider adding yoga or Pilates to improve flexibility, balance, and core strength while reducing stress.

Remember to consult with a healthcare provider before starting any new exercise program, especially if you have any medical conditions or concerns. Additionally, listen to your body and adjust the intensity of the exercises as needed.

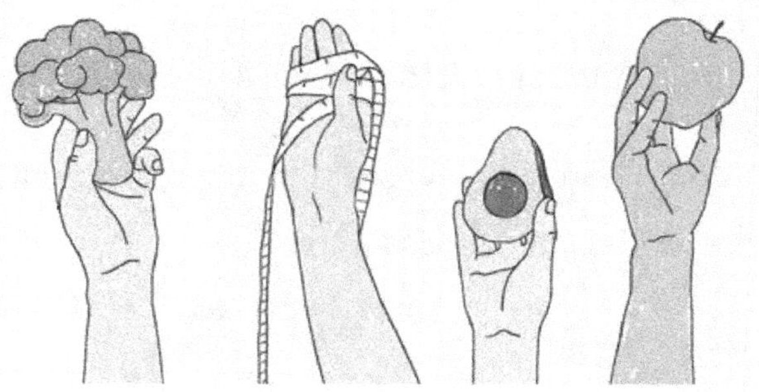

CHAPTER 7

Overcoming Challenges

Staying motivated and overcoming challenges during weight loss can be tough, but with the right mindset and strategies, it's absolutely achievable. Here are some tips to help you stay motivated and overcome common challenges:

Staying Motivated

Set Realistic Goals: Set achievable, realistic goals for yourself. Break down your larger goal into smaller, more manageable milestones. Celebrate each milestone you achieve.

Find Your Why: Understand why you want to lose weight. Whether it's to improve your health, boost your confidence, or have more energy to keep up with your kids, knowing your reasons will help you stay motivated.

Create a Support System: Surround yourself with supportive friends, family, or a weight loss group. Having people who cheer you on and hold you accountable can make a huge difference.

Track Your Progress: Keep track of your workouts, measurements, and food intake. Seeing your progress over time can be incredibly motivating.

Reward Yourself: Treat yourself when you reach your goals. Choose non-food rewards like a massage, a new workout outfit, or a fun activity.

Visualize Success: Picture yourself reaching your goals. Visualizing your success can help keep you focused and motivated, especially when times get tough.

Overcoming Challenges

Stay Consistent: Consistency is key. Even when you're not seeing immediate results, keep going. Progress takes time.

Deal with Setbacks Positively: Setbacks are a natural part of the process. Don't let them derail you. Instead, learn from them and use them as motivation to keep pushing forward.

Find Healthy Coping Mechanisms: Instead of turning to food for comfort, find other ways to deal with stress or emotions. Try activities like journaling, meditation, or going for a walk.

Avoid All-or-Nothing Thinking: Don't let one bad day ruin your progress. If you slip up, acknowledge it, and then move on. Every healthy choice you make is a step in the right direction.

Mix up Your Routine: If you're feeling bored or unmotivated, change up your exercise routine. Try a new workout class, go for a hike, or learn a new sport.

Focus on Non-Scale Victories: Remember that the scale isn't the only measure of success. Celebrate other achievements like increased energy, improved mood, or fitting into smaller clothes.

Get Back on Track Quickly: If you have a bad day or week, don't let it spiral out of control. Get back on track with your healthy habits as soon as possible.

Seek Professional Help if Needed: If you're struggling to stay motivated or overcome challenges, don't be afraid to seek help from a therapist, nutritionist, or personal trainer.

Remember, weight loss is a journey, and there will be ups and downs along the way. Stay positive, stay focused, and don't give up. You've got this!

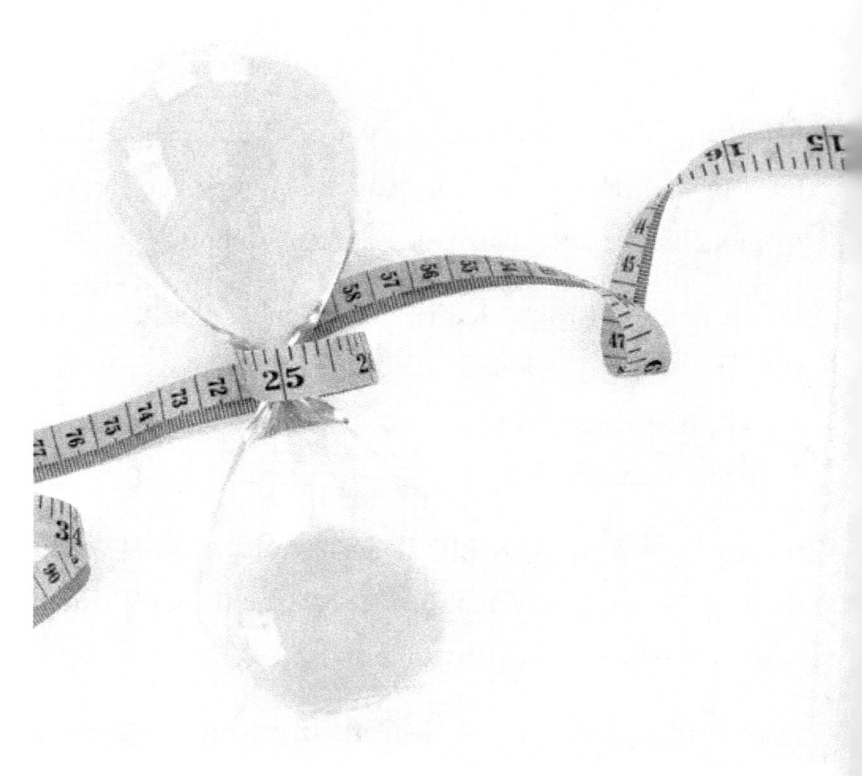

CHAPTER 8

Maintaining Your Weight Loss

Maintaining weight loss can be as challenging as losing weight in the first place. Here are some tips to help you maintain your weight loss and live a healthy lifestyle:

Establish Sustainable Habits:

- Aim for a balanced diet that includes plenty of fruits, vegetables, lean proteins, and whole grains.

- Practice portion control and mindful eating.

- Limit your intake of processed foods, sugary drinks, and unhealthy snacks.

- Cook more meals at home using fresh ingredients.

Stay Active:

- Continue with regular exercise even after you've reached your weight loss goals.

- Find physical activities that you enjoy and make them a part of your routine.

- Aim for a combination of cardiovascular exercise, strength training, and flexibility exercises.

- Set realistic fitness goals and challenge yourself to improve.

Monitor Your Weight:

- Weigh yourself regularly to track any changes.

- Keep a food diary to monitor your eating habits.

- Be aware of any changes in your body and address them promptly.

Practice Self-Compassion:

- Be kind to yourself and recognize that maintaining weight loss is a journey with ups and downs.

- Don't be too hard on yourself if you have setbacks.

- Celebrate your successes and focus on the positive changes you've made.

Build a Support System:

- Surround yourself with people who support your healthy lifestyle choices.

- Join a support group or find a workout buddy to keep you motivated.

- Share your successes and challenges with others who understand what you're going through.

Manage Stress:

- Find healthy ways to manage stress such as meditation, deep breathing exercises, or yoga.

- Avoid using food as a coping mechanism when you're stressed or emotional.

- Get plenty of rest and prioritize self-care.

Be Consistent:

- Stick to your healthy eating and exercise habits even after you've reached your goal weight.

- Remember that maintaining weight loss is a lifelong commitment.

Stay Hydrated:

- Drink plenty of water throughout the day to stay hydrated and avoid mistaking thirst for hunger.

- Limit your intake of sugary drinks and alcohol.

Plan for Challenges:

- Anticipate situations that may challenge your weight loss efforts, such as holidays or vacations.

- Plan ahead and make healthy choices whenever possible.

Seek Professional Help When Needed:

- If you're struggling to maintain your weight loss, consider seeking help from a registered dietitian, therapist, or weight loss support group.

- They can provide you with the tools and support you need to stay on track.

Maintaining weight loss requires commitment, consistency, and a willingness to make healthy choices every day. By adopting a balanced diet, staying active, managing stress, and seeking support when needed, you can successfully maintain your weight loss and live a healthier, happier life. Remember that small changes can add up to big results over time, so stay focused and keep moving forward.

CHAPTER 9

Frequently Asked Questions (FAQs):

Q: Will these recipes help me lose weight?

A: Yes, the recipes in this cookbook are designed to support your weight loss journey by providing nutritious, low-calorie meals that are satisfying and delicious. Each recipe includes calorie information and portion sizes to help you manage your intake.

Q: Are the ingredients easy to find?

A: Yes, the recipes in this cookbook use common ingredients that are easy to find at most grocery stores. You won't need to hunt for specialty items, making it convenient to follow these recipes.

Q: Are the recipes suitable for vegetarians/vegans?

A: Yes, we have included a variety of recipes suitable for vegetarians and vegans. You'll find plenty of plant-based meal options that are both nutritious and satisfying.

Q: Can I customize the recipes to fit my dietary needs?

A: Absolutely! Many of the recipes include substitution options to accommodate various dietary needs and preferences. Whether you're gluten-free, dairy-free, or have other dietary restrictions, you'll find options that work for you.

Q: How many servings do the recipes make?

A: Each recipe includes information on the number of servings it yields, along with portion sizes and nutritional information per serving.

Q: Will these recipes be suitable for my family?

A: Yes, these recipes are designed to be enjoyed by the whole family. They're not only healthy but also delicious and satisfying, making them perfect for family meals.

Q: Are the recipes time-consuming to prepare?

A: While some recipes may require a bit more time, many are quick and easy to prepare, making them perfect for busy weeknights. We've included a variety of recipes to fit different schedules and cooking skill levels.

Q: Are the recipes kid-friendly?

A: Yes, we've included plenty of recipes that are kid-friendly and sure to please even the pickiest eaters. From healthy versions of classic comfort foods to fun and flavorful snacks, there's something for everyone in the family to enjoy.

Q: Will these recipes help me maintain my weight once I've reached my goal?

A: Yes, these recipes are not only great for weight loss but also for weight maintenance. They focus on whole, nutritious ingredients that will help you stay satisfied and energized, making it easier to maintain a healthy weight long-term.

Q: Can I still enjoy my favorite foods while following these recipes?

A: Absolutely! We believe in balance and moderation, so you'll find healthy versions of your favorite foods in this cookbook. Whether you're craving pizza, pasta, or dessert, we've got you covered with delicious, guilt-free recipes.

Chapter 10: ACHIEVING LASTING SUCCESS

Congratulations on taking the first step towards a healthier, happier you! In this cookbook, we've provided you with a diverse range of delicious and nutritious recipes tailored specifically for women on a weight loss journey. We understand that embarking on this path can sometimes feel overwhelming, but rest assured, you're not alone. With the right tools, knowledge, and support, you can achieve your weight loss goals and live a more fulfilling life.

As you journey through these pages, here are some key points to keep in mind:

Balanced Nutrition: Each recipe in this cookbook is carefully crafted to provide the right balance of macronutrients, ensuring you get the energy you need while staying within your calorie goals. By choosing whole, nutrient-dense ingredients, you'll not only nourish your body but also support your weight loss efforts.

Variety and Flavor: Healthy eating doesn't have to be bland. We've included a wide variety of flavorful recipes to keep your taste buds excited and satisfied. From vibrant salads to hearty soups, and indulgent desserts to satisfying snacks, there's something for every craving and occasion.

Portion Control: While the recipes in this cookbook are designed to be nutritious and satisfying, it's essential to pay attention to portion sizes. Listen to your body's hunger and fullness cues, and practice mindful eating to enjoy your food more and prevent overeating.

Regular Exercise: While a healthy diet is a crucial component of weight loss, regular exercise is also essential for achieving and maintaining your goals. We encourage you to combine these nutritious recipes with a consistent exercise routine that includes cardiovascular exercise, strength training, and flexibility exercises for optimal results.

Consistency and Patience: It's important to remember that sustainable weight loss takes time and patience. There may be ups and downs along the way, but by staying consistent with your healthy eating and exercise habits, you'll gradually see progress and positive changes in your body and overall well-being.

With dedication, perseverance, and the right tools, you can achieve your weight loss goals and live a healthier, happier life. Remember, you're capable of more than you know, and we're here to support you every step of the way.

So, here's to you and your journey to a healthier, happier you! Here's to nourishing your body, fueling your soul, and embracing the incredible transformation that lies ahead.

Happy cooking, happy, healthy eating, and most importantly, here's to your success and well-being!

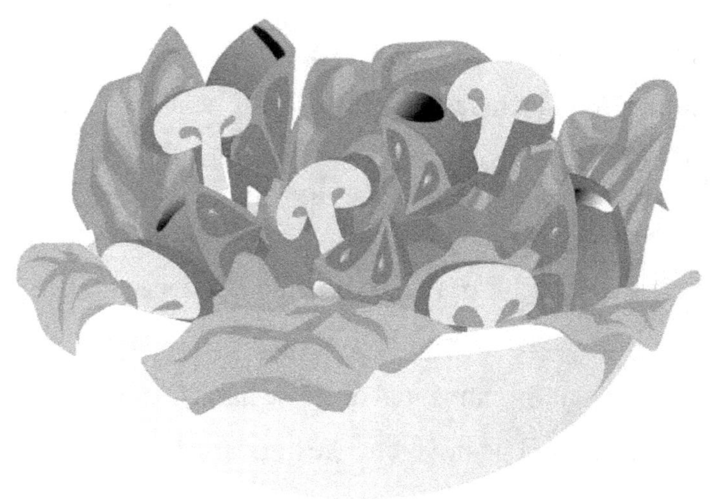

WEIGHT LOSS TRACKER

Date

Weight

Loss Gain

Notes

Date

Weight

Loss Gain

Notes

Date

Weight

Loss Gain

Notes

Date

Weight

Loss Gain

Notes

Date

Weight

Loss Gain

Notes

Date

Weight

Loss Gain

Notes

Date

Weight

Loss Gain

Notes

Date

Weight

Loss Gain

Notes

Date

Weight

Loss Gain

Notes

Date

Weight

Loss Gain

Notes

Date

Weight

Loss Gain

Notes

Date

Weight

Loss Gain

Notes

Date

Weight

Loss Gain

Notes

Date

Weight

Loss Gain

Notes

Date

Weight

Loss Gain

Notes

Date

Weight

Loss Gain

Notes

Date

Weight

Loss Gain

Notes

Date

Weight

Loss Gain

Notes

Date

Weight

Loss Gain

Notes

Date

Weight

Loss Gain

Notes

Date

Weight

Loss Gain

Notes

Date

Weight

Loss Gain

Notes

Date

Weight

Loss Gain

Notes

Date

Weight

Loss Gain

Notes

Date

Weight

Loss Gain

Notes

Date

Weight

Loss Gain

Notes

Date

Weight

Loss Gain

Notes

Date

Weight

Loss Gain

Notes

Date

Weight

Loss Gain

Notes

Date

Weight

Loss Gain

Notes

Date

Weight

Loss Gain

Notes

Date

Weight

Loss Gain

Notes

Date

Weight

Loss Gain

Notes

Date

Weight

Loss Gain

Notes

Date

Weight

Loss Gain

Notes

Date

Weight

Loss Gain

Notes

Date

Weight

Loss Gain

Notes

Date

Weight

Loss Gain

Notes

Date

Weight

Loss Gain

Notes

Date

Weight

Loss Gain

Notes

www.ingramcontent.com/pod-product-compliance
Lightning Source LLC
Chambersburg PA
CBHW050817250726
48653CB00006B/2266